EUTHANASIA

EUTHANASIA

Which "M" is it?
Mercy or Murder?

Zakyah Basri

authorHOUSE®

AuthorHouse™
1663 Liberty Drive
Bloomington, IN 47403
www.authorhouse.com
Phone: 1-800-839-8640

First published by AuthorHouse   01/12/2012

ISBN: 978-1-4678-8325-2 (sc)
ISBN: 978-1-4678-8326-9 (ebk)

Printed in the United States of America

Contents

"To all who may think of this moment as the start and as the bright light on their life—To others who may think about the end of this moment as the end of their suffering and the start of relieve . . . Yes, to all who ask for relieve. Bless you all."

Euthanasia

Which "M" Is It—

Mercy or Murder?

Chapter 1

Introduction

Chapter 1

Introduction

"Please do everything to save his life." It is always heard at any place where care is given, although it is not said in each and every situation. Nowadays, the doctor's decision about his or her patients has become a dilemma. Is it the doctor's duty to relieve pain and suffering even by taking the patient's life? Or should she or he respect human life and stand back, waiting for nature to take its course? Some people argue that in certain circumstances killing someone to relieve his or her suffering should be considered as a mercy killing, while others believe that letting someone die naturally is a matter of respecting human life.

That type of decision has been described by Boseley (2010) as an ethically controversial decision. A House of Lords Select Committee has defined euthanasia, which is an important issue in medical ethics, as the intentional intervention to end a life in order to relieve uncontrolled pain and suffering (Harris 2001). Euthanasia is an essential issue in today's world. However, it is still a negotiable question without any clear-cut answers.

This book presents a review of some of the literature about different countries' views on euthanasia. It illustrates some arguments about its types and the main causes with which we have to be concerned. Furthermore, it makes an argument about the pros and cons of different views—social, religious, financial, and medical.

In a very simple way this book will allow the reader to understand this issue and find his or her own opinion regarding this matter.

Chapter 2

Literature Review

Chapter 2

Literature Review

About 400 years B.C., Hippocrates, known as the Father of Medicine, said in his famous oath, "I will give no deadly medicine to any one if asked, nor suggest any such counsel." (Miles 2005)

The word "euthanasia" is a Greek word that means "good death". The term euthanasia was used by the historian Suetonius to describe how the emperor Augustus died quickly and without suffering in his wife's arms. In the seventeenth century, Francis Bacon was the first to use the word euthanasia in a medical context to describe an easy, happy, and painless death. He also referred to an "outward euthanasia", which related to a spiritual concept, the preparation of the soul (Dowbiggin 2003).

Then In 1870, Samuel Williams, who was a politician in the United States House of Representatives, was the first person to suggest the idea of using anaesthetics and morphine to deliberately end a patient's life. Over the next three decades, euthanasia was widely discussed in the United States and Britain. In 1906, an Ohio bill that would have legalized euthanasia was in the end defeated (Emanuel and Ezekiel 2004). In 1935, the Euthanasia Society of England was formed to support euthanasia (Otlowski 1997).

Four years later, the Nazis established a euthanasia program in Germany to end "life unworthy of life". In the beginning it was focused on new-borns and young children who showed signs of mental retardation, physical anomalies, or other symptoms, but later on it expanded to include the old, the terminally ill, and hopeless cases (George 1992).

In 1995, Australia's Northern Territory passed a bill that legalized euthanasia, but it was changed in 1997 by the Australian Parliament. In 1998 the state of Oregon legalized assisted suicide, and after that in 2000, the Netherlands became the first country in the world to legalize euthanasia.

Two years later, Belgium followed and became the second country (Cohen-Almagor 2005).

Over the years, euthanasia has been the target of the "slippery slope" argument. In addition, the conception of euthanasia has been changing as a result of changing policies and views. The historical view of euthanasia as a painless and quick death has changed. Nowadays, it tends to refer to the ending of a terminally ill patient's life, not necessarily by the patient's own decision. We must be concerned not only about the reason for euthanasia but also the way it is carried out.

Euthanasia has been widely debated and questioned without any clear answers emerging. Do we have the right to end our own life? What about the lives of others? Is it legal to do so?

Chapter 3

Types of Euthanasia

Chapter 3

Types of Euthanasia

To begin with, different forms of euthanasia have been classified in many different ways based on the way it is administered and who makes the decision.

Its administration is either passive or active. The main difference is that active euthanasia involves doing something to cause the patient's death. For instance, it could happen by using lethal injection in order to terminate someone's suffering and life. Passive euthanasia, on the other hand, means withholding an important treatment or procedure that might keep the patient alive (Harris 2001). Examples include withholding dialysis from patients with terminal-stage renal failure or withholding chemotherapy from cancer patients.

Regarding the other method of classification, "mercy killing" can be classified based on who is the one who decides to end the patient's life. There are three general types that fall into this category—voluntary, involuntary and non-voluntary euthanasia. Each of these is the subject of huge argument, particularly in terms of their eligibility.

First, voluntary euthanasia, which is also referred to as assisted suicide, is the subject of great controversy nowadays. It generally means applying death by the patient's choice and under the doctor's supervision or assistance. The latest research done by the National Centre for Social Research shows that eight out of ten of people support a change in the law to allow doctors to help patients who are terminally ill and want to die to end their lives (BBC Health News 2007). About 60% supported the view that doctors should be able to prescribe, but not administer, drugs to someone to end his or her own life. Around a third thought assisted suicide should be allowed in cases where the patient has severe illness, such as the terminal stage of renal failure, while only 24% agreed that euthanasia should be legal for someone who does not have terminal illness but is still in severe pain (BBC Health News 2007). However, voluntary euthanasia applied with the doctor's assistance would be considered murder

(Thomas and Terry 2009). Moreover, if it is done based on the patient's decision, it would be suicide. As we know, committing suicide is prohibited. In both interpretations, euthanasia tends to be a crime against human identity. West's *Encyclopedia of American Law* asserts that "a 'mercy killing' or euthanasia is generally considered to be a criminal homicide." (Cohen 2009)

But, why does a patient want to die? Is it the fear of suffering? Or is it a defect in the medical services? Is it really his or her decision, or is it the doctor's decision in the first place? There must be a reason which makes the person decide to end his or her life, but is she or he mentally healthy enough to make this type of decision? If all these questions have been answered and all these obstacles crossed, does the patient still want to die? If the answer is yes, this would be beyond our comprehension.

Therefore, many causes can be claimed to have incited the patient to make a decision about euthanasia or even to think about it. These include severe illness, fear of pain, depression, the advice of his or her doctor, and even insufficient healthcare. Most terminally ill patients who think about ending their lives are in severe pain. They might think about euthanasia as a last resort to eliminate and end their suffering and pain. In other words, some of them prefer to die rather than suffer.

Oregon's *Death with Dignity Act* summary in 2009 shows that people who choose an assisted death are always terminally ill. However, it is not always the situation that severely ill patients tend to end their lives. Patients with severe illness are expected to be sensitive and in need of any support which help them to face their difficult times. This type of help could be social or healthcare support. They might be thinking about dying as a way to run away from their situation. In other words, they need the empathy of others in order to get through difficult times with their diseases. They need to feel alive even if they are expected to die.

According to Campbell (2010), in her article "Disabled people need to live, not die", terminally ill and disabled patients were "not being heard" in this argument. This led to the formation of Not Dead Yet UK. She also says that most terminally ill patients might think about euthanasia because of their fear of pain, of losing their dignity, and of being a burden. All these fears might come from their depression. In fact, if someone has a feeling that he is a burden on his family, he will definitely be depressed and might think about suicide.

The second category is involuntary euthanasia. It simply means deciding when it is better for someone to be dead—for example, a patient who is in a vegetative condition and most likely will never recover. That is to say, it is taking someone's life without his or her consent. It could be done by the doctor, the family, or a court decision.

The case of Tony Bland case is an obvious example. In 1989 he was injured in the Hillsborough football stadium disaster, which made him suffer from a persistent vegetative state for around three years. In this condition, the patient is usually semi-conscious but not aware and is considered to be brain-dead. In 1993 the Airedale NHS asked the court to make it legal for them to withdraw Tony's treatment, including his tube feeding, in order to give him a peaceful death with dignity. Eventually, the court agreed and Tony passed away some days later (Watt 2000).

However, it does not usually happen that the court makes such a decision, which shows the law's instability when it comes to applying decisions related to ending a patient's life without his or her consent. An example is the case of

Frances Inglis. She was the mother of a son Tom, who was twenty-two years old and suffering from severe brain injury. The doctors recommended removing the food and water to end his life. Doing so would in fact have caused him to die, but only after many weeks and with great suffering. According to his mother, the court should have taken this decision before she took matters into her own hands. She made the decision to reduce her son's suffering, arguing that was better for her son to go to heaven rather than suffer hell on earth. In the end, the court found her guilty of murder and sent her to jail (Booth 2010). Obviously, the doctors did not take the mother's opinion into account regarding her son's condition. At the same time, she is the only one who should take such a decision.

The last type of euthanasia is non-voluntary euthanasia. It occurs when the patient cannot give consent regarding the ending of his or her life, as is the case, for example, with the new-born. Regarding this type of euthanasia, the Nuffield Council on Bioethics believes that most premature babies do not survive; researchers state that only 1% of these babies are able to leave the hospital alive. Therefore, Professor Margaret Brazier, Professor of Law in the University of Manchester where the committee guidelines were produced, said that babies born prior to 22 weeks should not be resuscitated because of their low likelihood of survival. She also said it is not always right to put such a patient in such stress and pain without any clear results. (*The Guardian* 2006) However, Watt (2000) argues that premature babies are still human beings who have the right to live. Their life is worth a chance at survival. Therefore, intentional killing does not seem moral for those who already at risk. Moreover, as humans, they still need to be cared for or to be given a chance to survive, no matter whether they are at risk or not.

Furthermore, a study done by University College London Hospital found that the survival rates for babies born between 22 and 25 weeks had increased from 32% to 71% between 1981 and 2000, which might be the result of the higher quality of neonatal care (Jones 2006). In fact, there are around 250 units in the United Kingdom offering neonatal intensive care, high dependency, and special care (*The Guardian* 2006). That is to say, improving the quality of care can be a solution, particularly for new-borns and children at risk, rather than thinking about subjecting them to euthanasia.

Now that the different types of euthanasia have been described, some pros and cons will be illustrated by explaining the impact of euthanasia in different views.

Chapter 4

Some Views Related to the Debate

Chapter 4

Some Views Related to the Debate

The Social View

First, we will consider the social view and will see that opinions differ widely regarding the morality of euthanasia. We will look at a survey that shows societies' views about euthanasia and its morality in countries all over the world. Some people who may choose euthanasia as a solution to their suffering state that euthanasia is one of their rights as humans to have a good death. Others believe that mercy killing seems to be a moral act in that it helps terminally ill patients to end their suffering. Moreover, it is a morally acceptable act because it can be universalised (BBC Ethics 2010). However, others argue that its ability to be universalised is an important factor but not a sufficient one to make euthanasia morally acceptable and a good rule (BBC Ethics 2010).

Another argument addresses the morality of passive and active euthanasia. Some argue that passive euthanasia is morally acceptable, because the cause of death is a disease, not a human, while active euthanasia is immoral, because the "agent of death" is a person and could in fact be the patient himself. However, not everyone accepts this distinction. Some argue that in both cases a human being is involved. Whether the person commits assisted suicide or is killed under medical advice, the two situations are equivalent. That is to say, if active euthanasia is morally unacceptable, then passive euthanasia should be unacceptable also.

In fact, most people believe that euthanasia can be ethically unacceptable under special circumstances. This is can be seen in the results of a survey done by World Values Survey in 2007 about the morality of euthanasia and its justifiability in developing countries and some Islamic and Asian countries. The survey was done by giving a scale answers form, classified from 1 to 10, with 1 meaning "never justifiable" and 10 meaning "always justifiable". The results shown in the graphs below:

Figure 1: OECD/Developed Countries

The Netherlands, which one of the countries where euthanasia is legal, scored more than 6 points, as did Denmark, Japan, New Zealand, Switzerland, Australia, France, and Sweden. That is to say, most of them agreed that euthanasia is justifiable. On the other hand, Ireland, Mexico, Portugal, South Africa, and Hungary think otherwise, scoring between 3 and 4 points, which means they do not agree as much as the other countries.

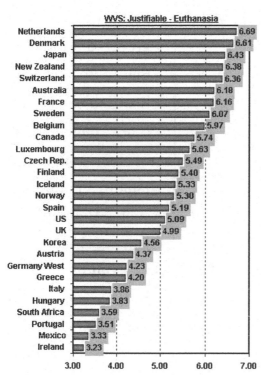

WVS: Justifiable - Euthanasia

Netherlands	6.69
Denmark	6.61
Japan	6.43
New Zealand	6.38
Switzerland	6.36
Australia	6.18
France	6.16
Sweden	6.07
Belgium	5.97
Canada	5.74
Luxembourg	5.63
Czech Rep.	5.49
Finland	5.40
Iceland	5.33
Norway	5.30
Spain	5.19
US	5.09
UK	4.99
Korea	4.56
Austria	4.37
Germany West	4.23
Greece	4.20
Italy	3.86
Hungary	3.83
South Africa	3.59
Portugal	3.51
Mexico	3.33
Ireland	3.23

Figure 2: Selected Asian Countries

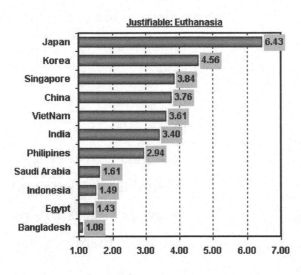

Japan is the only country among this group that agrees that euthanasia is justifiable. On the other hand, most of the Asian and Islamic countries, suchasBangladesh, Egypt, Indonesia, and Saudi Arabia, strongly disagree that euthanasia is justifiable. They scored less than 2 points. This is might be related to the religion factor (*World Values survey* 2007).

The Religious View

The second view is the religious view. This has a huge impact on the acceptability of euthanasia. Islam, Hinduism, Buddhism, and Christian beliefs and values vary towards euthanasia. However, Muslims, Jews, and Christians all believe that life is in the hand of God. He is the one who gives it to people, and he is the only one who can take it back. The next paragraphs present brief information about some of these religions and their values and beliefs regarding euthanasia.

To start with, Islam is the religion which is most opposed to any type of euthanasia. According to Boldly (cited in Smith 2006), "there is no place for euthanasia in Islam." (page 45) It is considered morally equivalent to suicide. Terminating human life is not the way to deal with suffering in Islam, but enduring the pain and suffering can be the way. Moreover, it could be the way towards a person's spiritual growth.

In Hinduism it is believed that birth, death, and rebirth constitute a cycle of recreation through many lives. This cycle should not be crossed. As a result, if things such as euthanasia take place, the person will have bad "karma" in his or her next life (Smith 2006).

Lama Rinpoche, a Buddhist philosopher, discussing Buddhist attitudes toward euthanasia, says that people cannot see the result of performing euthanasia. It cannot be obvious, even if the one who is doing it has a good motivation to euthanize a particular patient, such as to decrease his or her suffering. He also says that one of the results is that, while the patient might stop suffering in this life, she or he might suffer more in the other life. Therefore, euthanasia cannot be a good choice all the time (Rinpoche 2003).

Traditional Christian beliefs seem to be like the Islamic beliefs mentioned above. Christianity is opposed to euthanasia because life is a gift of God and has to be ended by him. Pope John Paul II described euthanasia as a type of culture of death and the manifestation of the social view of western societies which have abandoned the protection of life (Smith 2006).

So most religions' views are obviously opposed to euthanasia.

The Financial View

One of the reasons to support euthanasia stems from personal, family, and community economics (Smith 2006). There might be a difference between a patient who has to pay for his or her treatment and one who receives free healthcare services, which obviously will place the burden on the government economy. Therefore, some people argue that euthanasia might help cut healthcare spending. According to Smith (2003), the government might spend $40,000 in treating a terminally ill patient, whereas the cost to euthanize this same patient might be only $40. However, a study done in 1998 shows that, doctors' opinions could influence by this medical costs. That is to say, doctors who are cost-conscious and "practice resource-conserving medicine" are considerably more likely to write a lethal prescription for their severely ill patients *(Arch. Intern. Med.* 1998).

The Medical View

Doctors have different opinions regarding supporting euthanasia and changing the law. The result of a survey done among 4,000 doctors in the United Kingdom shows that one in every four doctors supports euthanasia. Moreover, around 35% of these doctors believed that mercy killing sometimes seems to be the only way to end patients' suffering and that therefore the law has to be changed (Devlin 2009).

However, some other doctors question how doctors can support euthanasia, when they know that it could not be effectively controlled by any law or policy. Herbert Hendin, who is the Executive Director of the American Suicide Foundation and Professor of Psychiatry at New York Medical College, asserts that Dutch euthanasia policies, as applied in Netherlands, are largely out of control. For example, as mentioned by Hendin (1997), "The alarming statistics in the Remmelink Report indicate that in thousands of cases, decisions that might or were intended to end a fully competent patient's life were made without consulting the patient." (page 77) He said that applying these polices does not seem to be validly acceptable, because it is not obviously the only solution to help terminally ill patients. According to him, palliative care could be another solution. It could be a key to supporting patients instead of giving them the option of ending their life. Joffe asserts that the solution for the majority of terminally ill patients' suffering is palliative care.

Chapter 5

Conclusion

Chapter 5

Conclusion

In conclusion, this book demonstrated that euthanasia has different pros and cons simply summarized in different views—social, religious, financial, and medical. Briefly, euthanasia could be a mercy killing for severely ill patients in order to end suffering. It could help in reducing many children's suffering and the rates of disabled children. It could be also one of the human rights for some people—to have a good death as well as a good life. It could be one of the ways of saving money in the health services or cutting government spending.

However, all people deserve to live, even if they have a terminal disease. They have a right to be cured, not to die. There are many different options to do that—supporting them emotionally and physically and giving them proper supportive palliative care, rather than euthanizing them. Although euthanasia seems to be acceptable in some societies, it is still avoided by many religions and beliefs. Furthermore, it is an unacceptable act under the medical ethics in many different countries, including the United Kingdom.

People, beliefs, spending, and health care are all different elements in this huge debate. Ultimately, it is difficult to predict everyone's opinion towards euthanasia. However, after reading this book, it might be less difficult to decide which "M" euthanasia is—Mercy or Murder.

References

References

Boseley, S. (2010), "Atheist doctors 'more likely to hasten death'". *The Guardian*, August 26 2010. Available on-line at:http://www.guardian.co.uk/society/2010/aug/26/doctors-religious-beliefs-terminally-ill.

Harris, N.M. (2001), "The euthanasia debate". J R Army Med Corps 147 (3): 367-70. PMID 11766225.

Miles, S.H. (2005), *The Hippocratic Oath and the Ethics of Medicine*. Oxford, Oxford University Press.

Dowbiggin, I. (2003). *A Merciful End: The Euthanasia Movement in Modern America.* New York, Oxford University Press.

Emanuel and Ezekiel J. (2004), "The History of Euthanasia Debates in the United States and Britain" in *Death and*

Dying: A Reader, edited by T. A. Shannon. Lanham, MD, Rowman & Littlefield Publishers.

Otlowski, M. (1997). *Voluntary Euthanasia and the Common Law*, New York, Oxford University Press.

George, A. (1992). "When Medicine Went Mad: Bioethics and the Holocaust" *The Nazi Doctors and the Nuremberg Code: Human Rights in Human Experimentation*, edited by George J. Annas and Michael A. Grodin. New York, Oxford University Press.

Cohen-Almagor, R. (2005), *Euthanasia in the Netherlands: The Policy and Practice of Mercy Killing.* USA, Springer Science + Business Media, Inc.

BBC Health News (2007), "Most support voluntary euthanasia". bbc.co.uk, 24 January 2007. Available on-line at: http://news.bbc.co.uk/1/hi/health/6293695.stm.

Thomas, J.G. and Terry, M.A., (2009), *Criminal Law* 10th edn. Belmont USA, Thomson Wadsworth.

Cohen-Almagor, R. (2009), "Belgian euthanasia law: a criticalanalysis".J.Med.Ethics35(7):436-439.doi:10.1136/jme.2008.026799. PMID 19567694.

Joffe, J. (2010). "A new proposal for assisted suicide". *The Guardian,* July 28 2010. Available on-line at: http://www.guardian.co.uk/commentisfree/belief/2010/jul/28/assisted-suicide-dying.

Campbell, J. (2010), "Disabled people need help to live, not die". *The Guardian*, June 3 2010. Available on-line at: http://www.guardian.co.uk/commentisfree/2010/jun/03/disabled-people-assisted-suicide.

Watt, H. (2000), *Life and Death in Healthcare Ethics: A Short Introduction.* London, Routledge.

Booth, R. (2010), "Mercy killer appeals against murder conviction for giving son fatal overdose." 21 July, *The Guardian*, July 21 2010. Available on-line at: http://www.guardian.co.uk/society/2010/jul/21/mercy-killer-appeals-son-heroin.

Jones, A. (2008), "Survival rates of premature babies static." *The Guardian*, April 12 2008. Available on-line at: http://www.guardian.co.uk/society/2008/apr/12/health. health.

Staff and Agencies (2006), "Extremely premature babies should be left to die, says report." *The Guardian*, November 15 2006. Available on-line at: http://www.guardian.co.uk/society/2006/nov/15/health.uknews.

BBC Ethics Guide (2010). "Arguments in favour of euthanasia." bbc.co.uk. Available on-line at: http://www.bbc.co.uk/ethics/euthanasia/infavour/infavour_1.shtml#h7.

Rinpoche, L.Z. (2003), *Advice and Practices for Death and Dying for the Benefit of Self and Others*. Portland, FPMT.

Smith, W. J. (2003), *Forced Exit: The Slippery Slope from Assisted Suicide to Legalized Murder.* USA, Spence Publishing.

Hendin, H. (1997), *Seduced By Death: Doctors, Patients and the Dutch Cure*. Washington, Norton and Co.

Devlin, K (2009), "One in three doctors support euthanasia." *The Telegraph*, March 25 2009. London, Telegraph Media Group Limited. Available on-line at: http://www.telegraph.co.uk/health/healthnews/5044885/One-in-three-doctors-support-euthanasia.html.